First Time Pregnant

Go from Clueless to Confident during Your First Pregnancy

Elane Holloway

CONTENTS

ELANE HOLLOWAY

INTRODUCTION

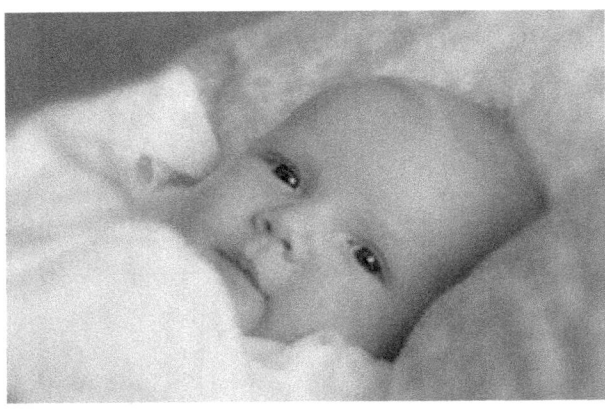

Congratulations! You're expecting a baby! This one of the most exciting and life-changing events in your, and perhaps even a little bit daunting. If this is your first pregnancy you have every right to be a little bit scared, but once you get over the minor discomforts of those first months and with the help of this book, you will be able to relax and enjoy every moment of this momentous time. This book is was designed for the first-time mother as a basic guide that will give you some of the most important and useful information about pregnancy and childbirth. The information an insightful tips will help you prepare yourself for the changes you will go through until you safely deliver your bundle of joy.

There are so many decisions to make when starting a family, especially upon learning that you're pregnant for the first time.

Our aim here is to arm you all the knowledge and advice you will need to take care of your health and your unborn baby's health during pregnancy, and be able to make informed decisions about your delivery.

In order to make informed decisions, it is very important for you to understand everything about pregnancy, and the changes you may expect to through both physically and mentally.

The first step to take when you first learn that you're pregnant is to consult a doctor immediately. The most common way a woman discovers that she is pregnant is when she misses a period, and takes an over-the counter pregnancy test. In some cases, a woman may not discover she's pregnant until she's well into the first few months, although this is quite rare. Whatever the case, the first thing your doctor will do is confirm that you are indeed pregnant and take it from there.

What is Antenatal care?

It is the monitoring of your health and your baby's throughout the term of your pregnancy until delivery by healthcare professionals. A woman's health and behavior affect the health and growth of the baby and certain illnesses may even put the baby's life at risk. It is therefore absolutely essential that you put yourself into the hands of a good doctor for antenatal care.

What to expect?

You will be given a series of appointments with a midwife or a doctor specialized in pregnancy (obstetrician OB/Gynecologist GYN.) Midwifes or nurses usually need a doctor on call for the delivery in case there are – God forbid - any complications during the birth. You may therefore choose a "shared" antenatal program where you alternate between a doctor and a midwife.

> **Pregnancy, labor and childbirth are life changing milestones in your life and should not be left to chance. A good doctor and excellent antenatal care are crucial**

If you are expecting your first child you may have up to ten antenatal appointments; if you've had a baby before you may only need about seven appointments. Remember that your individual situation may vary and will be the deciding factor on how often you need to see your doctor.

During each appointment you will go through some routine tests where you will be weighed, your blood pressure measured and a urine sample tested. Your doctor or midwife will confirm that you and your baby are well and also give you useful information about healthy eating, prescribe vitamins, give you exercise advice, answer your questions and discuss any fears you may have – in short, everything you need to ensure that you have a healthy pregnancy.

> **Important note: *If you prefer to deliver with the help of a midwife, Make sure your midwife is skilled and well-trained!***

On your first visit, your doctor or midwife will ask you some questions about your health and your family's health; they will also do some routine checks and blood tests so there's no need for alarm. The aim of these tests is to help ensure your safe pregnancy. You can expect the following:

One of the most important tests is that which is done to detect HCG (Human chorionic gonadotropin) which is a hormone that is produced during pregnancy, and which can be detected in blood or urine even before a missed period. More HCG is usually released in a multiple pregnancy such as twins or triplets than in a single pregnancy, and soon after delivery HCG will no longer be found in the blood.

At each of your antenatal appointments you will be asked to give a urine sample; this sample is checked for several things including albumen and protein. If they are found in the urine this means that you have an infection that needs to be treated.

You will be also be tested for HIV, the virus that causes AIDS, and if you are HIV positive both you and your baby will be given the treatment that reduces the risk of the baby being infected - HIV can be passed to a baby during pregnancy, at delivery, or after birth through breast feeding. Remember that it is very important to reduce the risk of transmission because one in five HIV-infected babies develop AIDS or die within their first year.

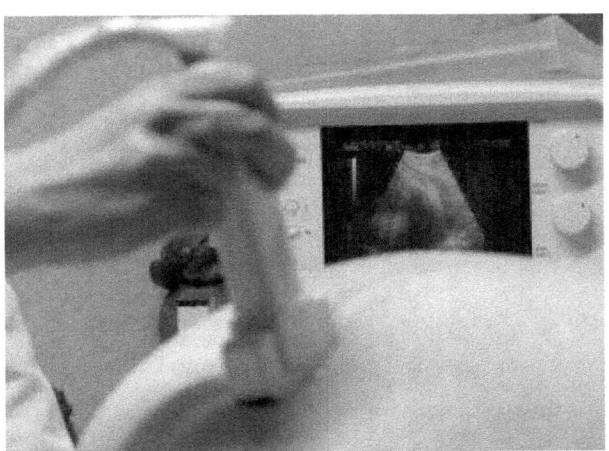

At the first visit you will also be given information about vitamin D supplements and folic acid (especially if the tests show that you're anemic, where you'll be prescribed acid and iron). Your doctor will also prescribe any other vitamin supplements you may need.

Your doctor will give you advice about sound nutrition, lifestyle factors such as smoking or drinking alcohol that might affect your health or the health of your baby.

You will be asked if you have had any complications in previous pregnancies.

Your midwife or doctor may also ask you about your job or your partner's job to see whether your work circumstances will affect your pregnancy or not. Certain jobs – such as working with chemicals – may be harmful and your doctor needs to be made aware of this

You will be asked about how you are feeling and whether you're feeling depressed. Your emotional health and wellbeing is also crucial and does affect your baby

Routine checks will include monitoring your weight, blood pressure, and your baby's heartbeats.

Knowing what to expect at your regular antenatal visits and being aware of the procedures should make you feel more comfortable and secure in the fact that you are doing your part to ensure the best for you and your baby's health.

Pelvic exams

If you've never had a pelvic exam before, you may be dreading this. Actually, even if you are accustomed to annual OB/GYN exams and pap smears, you'll probably still be dreading. Almost all women are very uncomfortable and nervous about the procedure, however, pelvic exams are very important for your health and that baby's. Some doctors allow a spouse or family member to be present with you during the exam so if this will make you feel more at ease, ask your doctor if this is possible. Some doctors do a pelvic exam on the very first visit than another one near the end of your pregnancy, usually at 36 weeks. Some doctors don't do pelvic exams at all! Your doctor will know best so just trust in him.

During a pelvic exam, the doctor will examine your cervix, uterus and fallopian tubes and ovaries. You will change into a hospital gown and will then get up onto the examining table and your feet will be put into stirrups. The doctor will begin the exam by checking your organs externally, pressing on your stomach. Next , he will use a speculum to begin the internal exam.

The internal exam allows the doctor to check for fibroids or any other abnormalities that may hinder the birth or any other abnormalities. He may also take cultures and fluid samples for certain tests and confirm how far along you are in your pregnancy, among other things. He may also do a pap smear.

The best way to relax is to take deep, slow breaths and to let your body go slack. tensing up will only make things more difficult for you and the doctor. Remind yourself that it will soon be over, pelvic exams take no longer than 10 minutes.

Don't miss appointments and assume that everything is fine as long as you are feeling well and you do not have any problems!

Relax! Your body knows exactly what it's doing and will prepare the perfect environment for your baby to grow and develop. Your antenatal visits are a an added insurance that everything's on the right track.

Choose a doctor or midwife you feel comfortable with. The emotional factor is equally important here and having a friendly and caring midwife or doctor will do wonders for those times when you're a bit under the weather. A patient healthcare professional who takes the time to listen, answer all your questions and calm your fears will make you less likely to miss your appointments.

Now let's move on

Symptoms and considerations during pregnancy

Pregnancy Symptoms vary from woman to woman; also because the early symptoms of pregnancy symptoms are often similar to what you experience during or before menstruation (sore breasts, fatigue, mild aches and cramps) they may sometimes not be recognized. In fact, seven out of ten women who are not actively planning to get pregnant only recognize these symptoms as signs of pregnancy by the time they are six weeks pregnant!

In this section of the book we shall discuss the most common symptoms of pregnancy, and considerations that should be made during that period.

Here is some of what you might experience during pregnancy, from nausea and fatigue to dizziness and mood swings to the various physical changes in your body:

The earliest symptoms of pregnancy include:

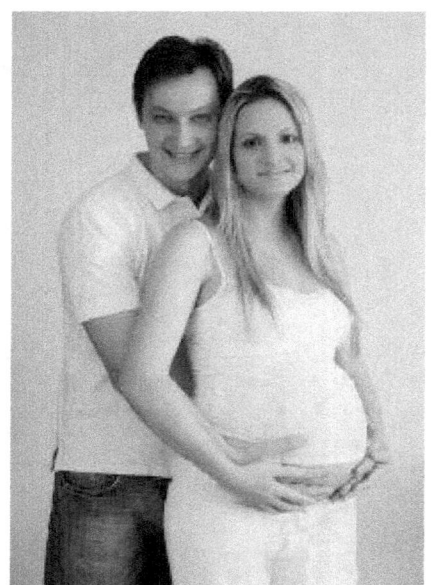

A missed period or irregular periods: If you are not actively trying to get pregnant, this symptom may go undetected for several week as is the case with many women.

Tender, swollen breasts: Hormonal changes such as the increased production of estrogen or progesterone which prepare the breasts for nursing will cause your breasts to swell and feel tender, sore or heavier.

Nipple changes: This has traditionally been a clear sign of pregnancy, where nipples may be deepen in color and the areola (the circular area around them) may also appear darker and enlarged. The veins in the breasts may also appear enlarged

If you have naturally small breasts, you will probably find these changes appealing – so make the most of your bigger, sexier breasts and take the opportunity to wear clothes that show off your natural cleavage! You may have to invest in larger-sized bras – but that's a trifling price to pay for your new – albeit temporary – curvy figure! Many women would agree that fuller breasts are one of the best perks of being pregnant.

While buying new bras you may want to invest in a few nursing bras as well if you are planning to breastfeed. A nursing bra is has special cups that are secured by hooks or snaps. The cups can then be unsnapped to expose the breast and allow the baby to nurse. Another style of nursing bra is made of lightweight, stretchy fabric that can be easily lifted up to expose the breast. Whatever your preference, They will make your task that much easier.

Tip: Be sure to buy and wear comfortable bras for during and after this period

Increased urination: This is the most common complaint by pregnant women; you will find yourself urinating more than usual and it may seem that you spend

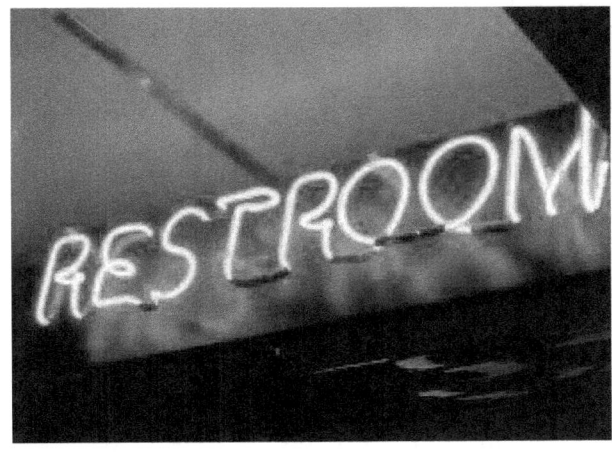

most of the time running to the bathroom! This is due to the enlargement in your uterus, which presses on your bladder. This is very normal, so DON'T WORRY! Feeling lie you have to use the bathroom every 5 minutes is a nuisance but otherwise it's a completely normal symptom.

Spotting: About eight to ten days before you would normally get your period, you might notice light spotting which is usually pinkish in color and not red like normal menstrual blood. Again, this is a common and normal symptom.

Feeling Sick: Nausea, often accompanied by vomiting and heightened sense of smell: this is the famous (or infamous) Morning sickness. It's the most common symptom of pregnancy, and I won't lie to you, it sucks. It's

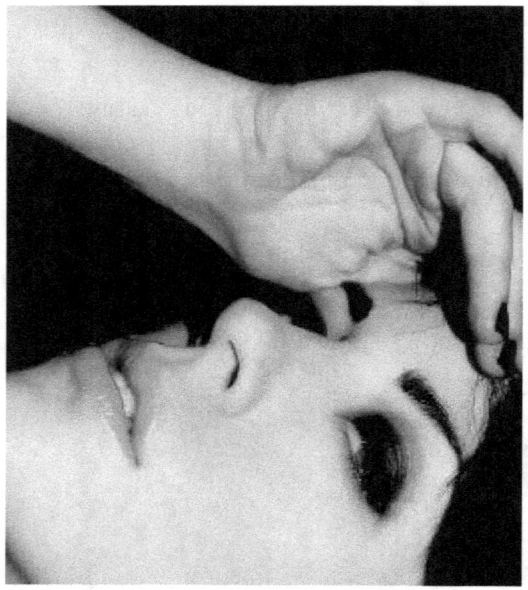

the most hated pregnancy symptom by women the world over.

Morning sickness can start as early as four weeks into pregnancy but most commonly starts in the sixth week. It includes feeling so nauseous that you actually vomit, and the sight of certain foods or a certain smell can also trigger it. The term "morning sickness" is deceiving. It can strike at any time of the day or night. Pregnancy hormones play a role in causing nausea during pregnancy. That's why you might find that certain smells that never bothered you before can actually make you vomit!

> ### The term "morning sickness" is deceiving. It can strike at any time of the day or night.

There are a few lucky women who breeze their pregnancy with very little to no morning sickness at all, and if you're one of those blessed few, congratulations!

Fatigue: During pregnancy a large amount of your body's energy is directed into building a life-support system for your baby, so your body is working harder to produce more quantities of certain hormones. One of these hormones is the progesterone which is a natural depressant of the central nervous system. This is why you may feel worn out and sleepy. Your body is also working hard to supply blood and nutrients to the baby which will also make you feel more tired.

Extreme fatigue can also be caused by anemia, so it's very important to eat iron-rich foods or take iron supplements. If this is the case, seek advice from your health professional. Again, this is a common symptom and no cause for worry; Try to make more time for naps and little rests throughout your day.

Bloating and constipation: Again, this is due to an increase in the progesterone hormone which slows digestion. Constipation may become a serious issue for some women as straining during bowel movements can cause hemorrhoids.

My best advice for reducing these symptoms is by drinking lots of water which helps ease constipation and bloating; try to drink 6- 8 glasses of water a day to ease constipation. Drinking lots of fruits juice (especially prune juice) is another healthy natural remedy. Increasing your dietary fiber by eating lots of fresh fruits and vegetables; not only are they great for constipation but are also packed with upper healthy nutrients for you and your baby.

Gentle exercise such as swimming, walking or yoga is another great way to reduce these symptoms. The good news is that constipation disappears fairly soon after you deliver your baby.

Hunger pangs and unusual cravings: Your body during pregnancy needs about 300 extra calories a day. Some women feel hungry all day long while others may find themselves craving for certain foods during pregnancy, especially foods that provide energy and calcium such as milk, cheese or meat. Some women may also notice a sudden distaste for foods they previously used to like.

Headaches: Headaches may occur frequently during pregnancy due to increased blood circulation caused by hormonal fluctuation. If you've gone cold turkey on smoking and caffeine after learning that you're pregnant, you may also experience headaches.

These types of headaches are called tension headaches; you will experience a squeezing pain or a dull ache on both sides of your heads. If you have headaches during your first trimester, you will find that they will disappear completely in your second trimester what your hormones stabilize.

Do not take any medication for headaches before consulting your doctor. You may also resort to natural headache relievers such as cold compresses, showers, relaxation techniques. Some women who suffer from debilitating headaches may resort to acupuncture.

Mood swings: This is a biggie and perhaps one of the most famous symptoms associated with pregnancy. Many women go through a spectrum of emotions and mood swings during pregnancy. Again, this is due to the immense changes happening in your body. Pregnancy is a wonderful life-changing experience but it can also be a very stressful time for you; it's only normal that you should have fears and concerns in addition to your joy at becoming a new mom. – all of this can lead to a rollercoaster of emotions.

You may find yourself liable to cry more easily than usual, or perhaps get upset over the slightest thing. Prepare your partner for these mood swings as he will most likely have to near the brunt of them!

Mood swings are more pronounced during the first trimester and then again during the last trimester when your body begins preparing for birth.

Strange cravings: Food cravings are a fact of pregnancy and are again associated with hormonal changes. You mustn't always give in to these cravings as they may lead to more weight gain then is healthy. Food cravings may range from none to moderate to outright bizarre. Some of the weirdest cravings experienced by women include ice, raw onion and fried eggs with mint sauce.

There is also another type of craving called 'pica' in which women crave non-food substances such as coal, soil, talcum powder, or soap among others. In certain areas of the world women actually so consumes these things but needless to say they can be harmful. If you experience pica cravings, speak to your doctor about them. He will be able to find out if you're getting the essential vitamins you need.

> **Britney Spears confessed that she had a craving for fried chicken throughout her pregnancy – with a big side helping of fresh soil!**

Scientists have found that eating a big nutritious helps curb cravings by up to 50%, so you may want to try that before putting "soil" on your grocery list!

Warning: Raw fish, meat and poultry are an absolute no-no no matter how strong your craving may be. They can be very harmful to you and your baby, as we'll explain later.

Heartburn and indigestion: If you are experiencing these symptoms then it is recommended that you avoid eating just before going to bed, avoid fatty foods, spicy foods, alcohol and caffeine, wear loose clothes, and always consult your doctor before taking any antacids.

Many women begin experiencing heartburn during the second half of pregnancy, and it comes and goes until they give birth. Avoid foods that can cause or increase heartburn such as carbonated drinks, citrus fruit, mustard, tomatoes, fried foods, processed meats and vinegar.

If you experience heartburn, try some of these natural heartburn-fighting foods that will give you relief:

- Bananas

- Apples

- Buttermilk

- Potatoes

- Fat-free cheeses

- Multi-grain bread

- Carrot or banana bread

- Brown rice

Leg cramps: Up to half of pregnant women experience leg cramps which usually occur at night. This is due to your weight gain as well as the uterus pressing down and constricting blood vessels in the lower region of the body. You can do the following to alleviate this condition:

- Wiggle your toes and rotate your ankles while sitting.

- Try to take a daily short walk; even 10 minutes is enough.

- Wear support stockings.

- Lie on your left side to improve circulation.

- Don't sit with your legs crossed.

- Have your spouse massage your feet and ankles before bed

If the cramps become too troublesome then you will have to discuss with your doctor the option of taking magnesium lactate or citrate in the morning and evening. If the cramps are accompanied be tenderness or swelling in the legs, call your doctor immediately.

ELANE HOLLOWAY

Considerations during pregnancy

There are a number of things that should be taken into considerations to ensure your health and well-being as a mother-to be as well the health of your baby.

These concern diet, lifestyle, and mental & emotional health.

A healthy diet, exercise, and plenty of rest are essential for your health during pregnancy

Certain foods should be avoided – not matter how strong your cravings - such as raw seafood, undercooked meat and deli meats which can be contaminated with salmonella and other toxins.

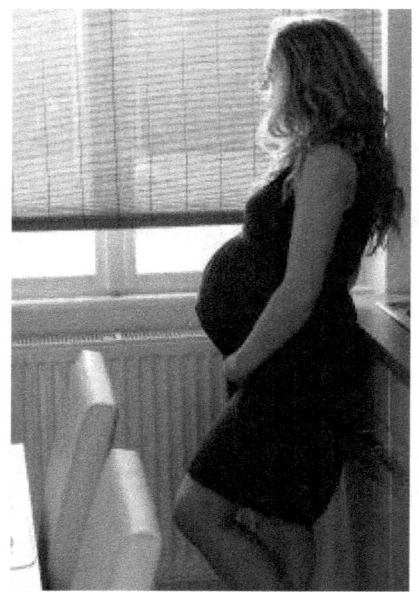

You don't really need me to tell you this but here goes - avoid smoking. The dangers of smoking for pregnant women have been well documented. If you're a smoker, stop immediately. Weight the discomforts of going cold turkey against the risks to your unborn child – mot a difficult choice, is it?

Avoid being a passive smoker as well, and stay away from drugs which can have a damaging effect on your baby.

If you believe you are experiencing pre-natal depression and not just normal mood swings, then you should seek help as soon as possible because your untreated depression can have harmful effects on the development of your baby.

Ask your partner, family, and friends to monitor your situation and help as much as they can.

Contradictory to the popular thought that women tend to suffer more from postnatal depression, studies have shown that rapid hormonal changes during pregnancy can disrupt brain chemistry and lead to depression. The following are warning signs that indicate prenatal depression:

- A feeling of deep sadness or emptiness throughout the day.

- Not being able to enjoy or find fun in activities you used to like.

- Extreme tiredness or fatigue, a feeling of listlessness.

- Extreme irritability and crying fits

- Inability to concentrate.

- Sleep disruption – you either sleep too little or too much.

- Feeling hungry and wanting to eat all the time.

- A feeling of hopelessness and unworthiness.

If you experience three or more of these symptoms for over a week, it's time to talk to your doctor about suitable treatment. If left untreated, prenatal depression can affect your baby's growth and may even lead to premature birth.

Exercise is so important during and after pregnancy that I can't recommend it enough. It boosts your spirits and can help you get over depression, but it is also very important for you to pay close attention to the signs your body is sending during exercise.

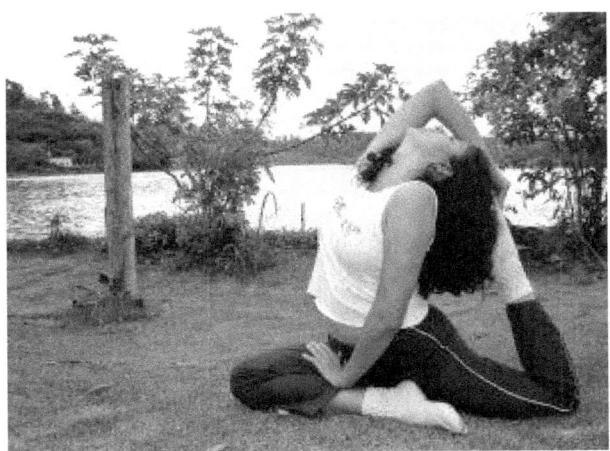

Yoga, swimming, and brisk walking are good exercise choices for pregnancy.

Avoid over-heating which can be very dangerous during pregnancy, so always make sure you exercise in the early morning, in the evening or in an air-conditioned gym to avoid over-heating which can cause dehydration, which in turn can cause dangerous complications. Always wear loose, comfortable clothing that will help to keep you cool while exercising.

Be sure to drink lots of water, not less than eight glasses per day.

Avoid over-exertion! Stop exercising immediately if you exceed the maximum recommended heart rate which is 140 beats per minute and wait until your heart beat slows down and returns back to its normal rate.

If you notice the following symptoms during exercising then these are signs for you to stop physical activity immediately and seek medical help:

- Dizziness.

- Chest pain.

- Increased heart rate.

- Vaginal bleeding or fluid leakage.

- Headache.

- Shortness of breath.

Avoid wearing high heels so you can walk more easily without falling! Comfortable low heeled shoes are will also be easier on your back once you start getting bigger.

Guidelines for good health:

Nutrition

You don't really need too many extra calories during pregnancy, especially in the first six months, while you will need an extra 200 - 300 calories a day in the last three months, so there's no need to "eat for two" as many people will wrongly advise you!

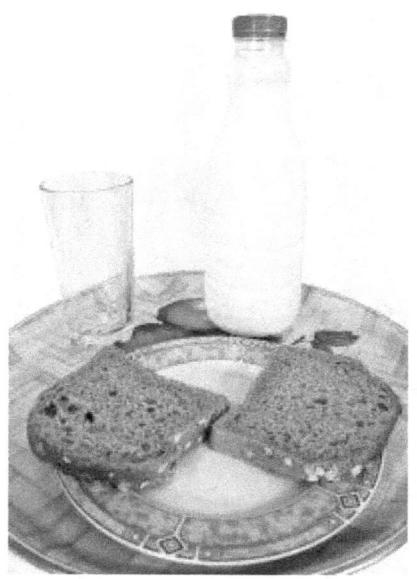

Eat a healthy and balanced diet whenever you can, which should consist of the following:

Keep up your energy levels with healthy snacks! Granola bars, nuts and dried fruits and freshly-made smoothies are ideal energy-boosters. Avoid junk food and excessive sweets!

Plenty of carbohydrates such as rice or bread; use them as bases for your meals. It is better to eat whole grain carbohydrates rather than white because they give you plenty of fiber.

At least five portions of vegetables and fruit daily.

Daily servings of protein of a minimum of 75 grams such as milk, eggs, nuts, and fish which is packed with vitamin D and omega-3 fatty acids - important for the development of the baby's nervous system! So try to have fish twice a week.

The top 10 best foods during pregnancy

1-	All colorful Fruits and veggies
2-	Lean meat
3-	Salmon
4-	Yoghurt
5-	Leafy greens
6-	Walnuts
7-	Salmon
8-	popcorn and whole wheat products
9-	Eggs
10-	Sweet potatoes

If you are worried about not eating well, you can take a vitamin supplement, but bear in mind that vitamin supplements aren't a total substitute for a balanced diet.

Use fish oil supplements if you don't eat fish. Make sure to use a supplement made from the body not from the liver of the fish (such as cod liver supplements) because fish liver oils contain a form of vitamin A which is not recommended during pregnancy.

Your supplement should contain 400 micrograms of folic acid which is essential in the first three months of pregnancy, and 10 micrograms of vitamin D which is important for your baby's future bone health.

If you have trouble swallowing your supplement, you can choose a chewable supplement or one in a powdered form that can be mixed with water.

Some foods are not safe to eat during pregnancy. I mentioned before raw seafood and undercooked meat; add to that undercooked ready-made meals which might contain a type of bacteria called Listeria. This is a bacteria which 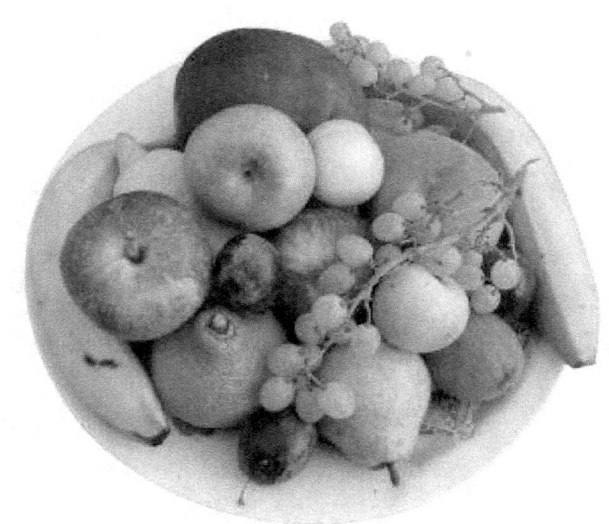 causes an infection called Listeriosis that may cause miscarriage. Listeria bacteria is destroyed by heat so if you should consider eating undercooked ready-made meals make sure to heat them thoroughly.

Avoid eating under cooked poultry as well because you can catch Salmonella which can cause food poisoning. Cook eggs well until both the white and yolk are firm.

Avoid the risk of catching Toxoplasmosis, an infection caused by a parasite that can affect your unborn baby. Wash your vegetables and fruits thoroughly to remove dirt, cook meat well, and wear gloves when handling garden soil and cat litter.

Too much caffeine may increase your risk of miscarriage, or having an underweight baby. 200 mg of caffeine per day (the equivalent of two mugs of instant coffee) won't harm your baby so stick to that.

If you are suffering from morning sickness, nausea or vomiting, the following tips will help you:

- Avoid fatty or spicy foods.

- Drink lots of fluids outside of mealtimes.

- Try to minimize odors while cooking by opening a window, for example.

- Eat small portions of food throughout the day rather than one big meal.

- If you are suffering from heartburn, eat lots of dairy products such as yoghurt, milk or buttermilk which really helps to relieve the symptoms and is super nutritious as well.

- Give up alcohol for your entire pregnancy! It could cause physical defects, emotional problems, central nervous system and brain damage in children. It simply is not worth the risk.

Finally, let me close with this tip again - This one is so important that I can't stress it enough - STOP SMOKING! Smoking can cause serious problems for you and your baby such as an increased risk of miscarriage, low birth weight or premature birth, so it's better to be safe than sorry!

Exercising

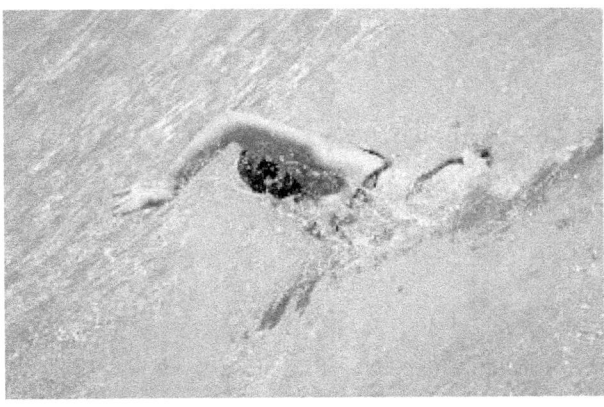

Until only a few decades ago it was believed that exercise was dangerous for mother-to-be. A pregnant woman needed to avoid as much activity as she could, and move and walk slowly. Today we know better, and health experts can't say enough about the benefits of exercise during pregnancy.

Most pregnant women can really benefit from exercising during their pregnancies. The idea that exercise is harmful to an expectant mother is an old wives tale; the reality is that regular mild exercise exercising is a big plus for you and your baby in many ways. The benefits include:

Look better: Increase the natural radiance of pregnancy with regular exercise, which improves the blood flow to your skin and body; you will simply glow with health and beauty.

Feel Better: Exercise boosts your energy level and gives you a great sense of wellbeing by releasing endorphins. Endorphins are chemicals in the body which react with the brain and give you a "natural high", a feeling of well-being and positivity

Prevents wear and tear on your joints, as they become lax during pregnancy as a result of hormonal changes.

It increases muscle strength.

It can help you sleep better as it relieves the stress and anxiety that could make you restless at night.

It reduces constipation and relieves backaches and other discomforts.

It helps you regain your pre-Pregnancy body more easily and quickly, by preventing excess weight gain and keeping your muscles toned.

It can lower your risks of complications, for example, gestational diabetes.

It will help prepare your body and muscles for birth, as it will help you control your breathing which can help you manage pain better.

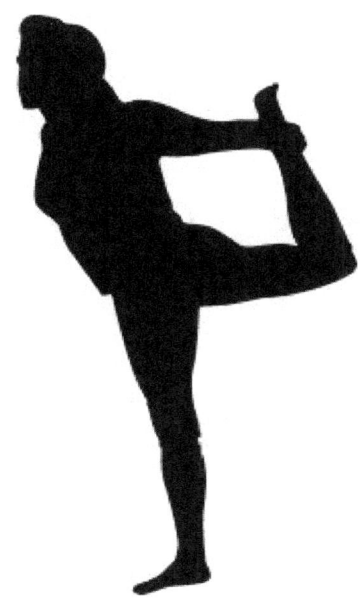

If you used to exercise regularly before you became pregnant, continue your programs but with modifications as needed.

If you were out of shape before becoming pregnant, don't give up! What better time to start getting fit than during this time when the exercises are not too strenuous. And once you see and feel the benefits, you're more likely to fit a regular workout into your schedule on a permanent basis.

It is very important to consult your doctor about exercising before you continue your old exercise routine or begin a new one.

Your doctor might advise you to limit your exercise or forego it altogether if you have:

- Vaginal bleeding.

- High blood pressure.

- Early contractions.

- Some forms of lung and heart disease.

- Very low iron levels (severe Anemia).

- If you were overweight or underweight before you were pregnant.

- If you are expecting twins.

These are somewhat rare cases and generally, the majority of expectant mothers benefit from exercise.

Exercise guidelines and tips

How long and how often?

The American College of Obstetricians and Gynecologists recommends has found exercising to be so beneficial for pregnant women that they recommend 30 minutes a day most days of the week (4-5 days). Again, this may depend on your fitness level and if you have been exercising regularly before pregnancy.

If you're new to exercise, start out with 2-3 days a week of 10-minute workouts, building up to the full 30 minutes then increasing the number of exercise days.

What type of exercise?

The ideal workout I one that gets your heart pumping, keeps your weight under control, keeps you agile and limber, manages weight gain, and prepares your muscles doe childbirth. Not all exercises are suitable for women pregnant women, such; the aim is to get the most benefit without putting physical stress on you or the baby.

Guidelines for exercising

-If you haven't exercised for a while, start small and gradually build up, as we mentioned before. Begin with five minutes of physical activity a day, and then build up to ten minutes, then fifteen and so on until you reach thirty minutes a day.

If you exercised regularly before pregnancy, you can continue to exercise at the same level while you are pregnant as long as you are feeling good, and your doctor finds it O.K.

Never exercise to the point of exhaustion or breathlessness. Pushing yourself too hard forces your body to use up oxygen that should be going to your baby.

What are the best exercises recommended during pregnancy?

Walking: A great for beginners; a relaxing nature walk or mild hike not only gives your legs and lower body a good workout, it also bathes you in a sense of wellbeing and serenity. If you're lucky enough to live near the beach, all the better for you – can there be a more perfect and relaxing walk?

Swimming: health and fitness experts see swimming as one of the best exercises pregnant mothers. Swimming is a great non-strenuous exercise that works large groups of muscles simultaneously. The weightlessness in the water is also ideal for expectant mothers carrying more than their normal weight.

Stationary bike: cycling on a stationary bike much safer for pregnant women than normal cycling, where you may need to swerve suddenly or hit a bump in the road.

Low impact aerobics: Aerobic exercise is the ideal cardiovascular workout for an expectant mother. Not only does it strengthen you heart but also tones and firms up the body, making it much easier for you to get back into full shape after the birth. Consider signing up for a special class for pregnant women (These have become quite common and can be found in almost any city). What a great way to work out as well as to chat and enjoy the camaraderie of other moms to be! An added benefit of working out under a certified instructor is that you can be sure that every move is safe for you and your baby.

Dancing: Another great exercise for getting that heart rate up. Join up for a dance class or enjoy dancing to your favorite tunes in the comfort of your own living room. Just make sure you avoid routines that require jumping or twirling.

> *Avoid overheating! Make sure to drink lots of fluids to stay hydrated.*

Tips for exercising safely:

Monitor your pulse and make sure that your heart rate doesn't exceed 140 beats per minute.

If you feel dizzy, weak, or have blurred vision stop exercising immediately and sit down and rest.

If you don't feel better within a few minutes after you stop exercising, call your doctor.

If your baby's movements appear to slow down or stop, take a rest.

Exercises to avoid during pregnancy

The American Pregnancy Association strongly advises against the following sports and exercises during pregnancy, even in the first trimester when you may not be certain that you're pregnant at all:

- Any sports that could result in falls you fall such as horseback riding, skiing, diving, or skating.

- Collision sports such as tennis or squash are not recommended due to the risk of being hit in the stomach, as well as slipping and falling.

- Contact sports such as basketball, volleyball and soccer.

- Extreme sports such as skateboarding, bike tricks and motocross, bungee jumping and surfing.

Any sport with a high injury or fall rate puts your baby's life at risk.

Tips:

When you reach the sixteenth week of pregnancy skip exercises that include lying flat on your back or standing in one place for a long time, as these types of exercises can reduce the blood flow to your baby.

Always remember to wear good shoes and watch your balance - and don't forget that your center of gravity has changed.

Exercise doesn't have to be formal to have beneficial effects; any activity that you can do every day such as walking, or doing housework counts.

If you have other young children and simply no time to exercise, consider an energizing, brisk walk with a push chair, or exercise along with a DVD during your kids' naptime.

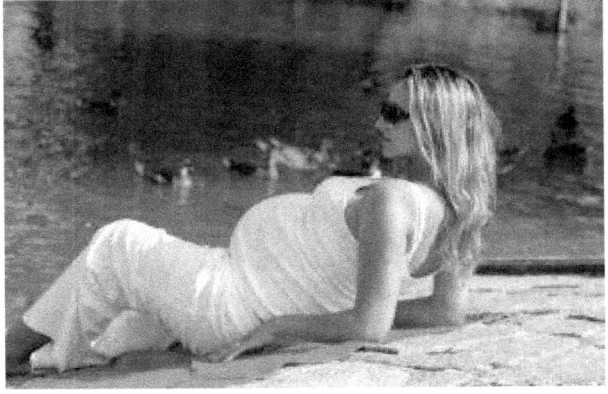

Lifestyle

Your lifestyle considerations during pregnancy should be geared to towards getting you through the next 9 months comfortably and smoothly with the maximum health benefits for you and your baby.

The pregnancy Lifestyle includes various factors ranging from the food you eat, exercise, medication/ supplements, the amount of sleep you get, to the level of stress you experience daily.

Here are some of the factors you need to consider in your lifestyle:

Good Nutrition

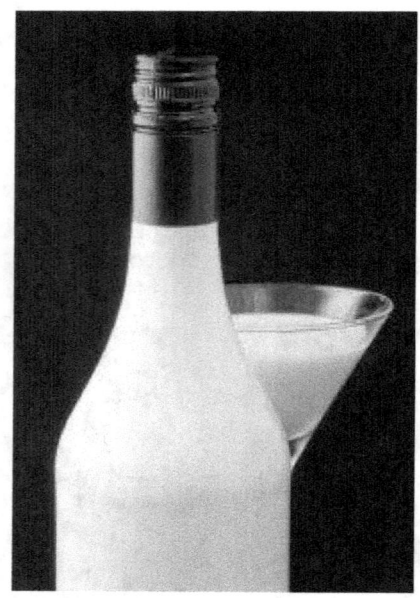

Food requirements change during pregnancy. pregnant women should eat body building foods, health protective foods, and energy boosting foods.

Avoid over-nutrition or under nutrition during pregnancy as both of them can create serious health risks for you and your baby. Also, remember what we mentioned before: gorging yourself because "you're eating for two" is not the way to go. Moderate but highly nutritious food portions are the best gif you can give to your baby during this time.

Use iodized salt.

Eat only well cooked fish, meat, and eggs.

Avoid low energy diets.

The following is a list of super-healthy, must-eat foods for expectant mothers. Make sure to include them in your diet:

- Calcium-rich dairy products

- Whole grains such as whole wheat breads and cereals, pasta and brown rice.

- Beans – all types of beans; white beams, black beans, pinto beans, black-eyed peas, chickpeas and lentils are an excellent source of protein. A large number of women go off meat during pregnancy as it makes then nauseous, and beans are an excellent and more palatable alternative and can be prepared in many appetizing ways.

- Salmon, which is packed with super healthy Omega-3 fatty acids. Just make sure you grill or broil it.

- Berries are an excellent source of nutrition and also contain antioxidants.

- Yoghurt: prepare a delicious and super healthy snack by chopping a banana (or other fresh fruit of your choice) into a container of plain yoghurt. A cold yoghurt smoothie also makes a refreshing drink on hot summer days, and is healthier than a cola or soft drink.

- Eggs – again make sure they are well-cooked. Avoid poached eggs during the term of your pregnancy.

Smoking and passive smoking

In addition to stopping smoking, avoid being a passive smoker during pregnancy in order to prevent an increased risk of pregnancy complications, premature birth, sudden infant death syndrome (SIDS), Asthma and upper respiratory tract infections.

A smoke-free pregnancy is best for you and your baby, so if your partner, family members or guests in your home are smokers, don't be hesitant about banishing them to the back yard or to a balcony when they want to light up.

If you happen to be a smoker yourself, here are some tips to help you stop smoking during your pregnancy – and hopefully for good!

Make a list of the reasons you want to stop and refer to them whenever you feel like smoking. In this case, a healthy, bouncing baby should be at the top of that list!

It is usually best to stop once and for all. I've found that a lot of women stop cold turkey the minute they find out they're pregnant. The fear of harming their unborn baby far outweighed any

Ask friends and family members to help by giving you emotional support.

Get rid of ashtrays and all cigarettes.

Don't worry if you experience withdrawal symptoms like headaches, nausea, anxiety, or just feeling awful when you stop smoking. Remember, you're doing this for your baby's health! These symptoms will gradually ease after two to four weeks.

Think positive! After a few weeks you will smell better, cough less, and have more money!

Caffeine: Make sure you don't have more than 200 mg of caffeine a day as high levels can cause low birth weight and in some cases even miscarriage. Use the following guide to calculate your caffeine intake:

Product	Amount of caffeine
I cup of coffee	75 mg
1 mug of coffee	100 mg
1 cup of tea	50 mg
1 mug of tea	75 mg
Plain chocolate – 1 50-gm bar	50 mg
1 can of energy drink	80 mg

Some cold and flu medicines also contain caffeine and should not be taken before consulting your doctor.

Medications/Drugs

You should check with your doctor if you are taking any medications during your pregnancy to find out if it is safe, or maybe he could give you another medicine that could be safer to use.

Don't hesitate to talk with your doctor if you are taking any illegal drugs and be sure that this information will be kept confidential.

It is better if you stop these drugs because you could be placing your baby at risk of premature birth, miscarriage, learning defects, and lots of other problems, so try to get help immediately.

Alcohol: For the sake of your baby stop drinking alcohol as it can cause damage to your baby which includes brain damage, and a low birth weight baby.

The work environment

Certain jobs may cause a risk to pregnancy, for instance:

- If you are a healthcare worker this may put you at a risk of contracting hepatitis B, or C so you must be immunized against this virus.

- If you work with chemicals or radiation, this may be toxic to an unborn baby.

- If you work with animals; for example if you work with lambs then you should avoid contact with them at lambing time because some of them are born contaminated with bacteria such as listeria, and toxoplasma which may harm your unborn baby.

- Also avoid cleaning cat litter because cat feces often carries toxoplasma bacteria.

In short, if you think that your job might put you at risk during your pregnancy then you should discuss this with your employer before you get pregnant.

Sleep and Rest

Try to get more sleep during your pregnancy, the best comfortable sleep position as recommended by doctors is by lying on your side with your knees bent and putting a pillow between your knees to decrease the strain on your lower back, this position also makes things easier on your heart and lungs, it also reduces constipation because it allows for better circulation.

You can put extra pillows behind your back and under your stomach to give you more support.

You can find special pregnancy pillows at many stores which are designed especially to support your body and stomach.

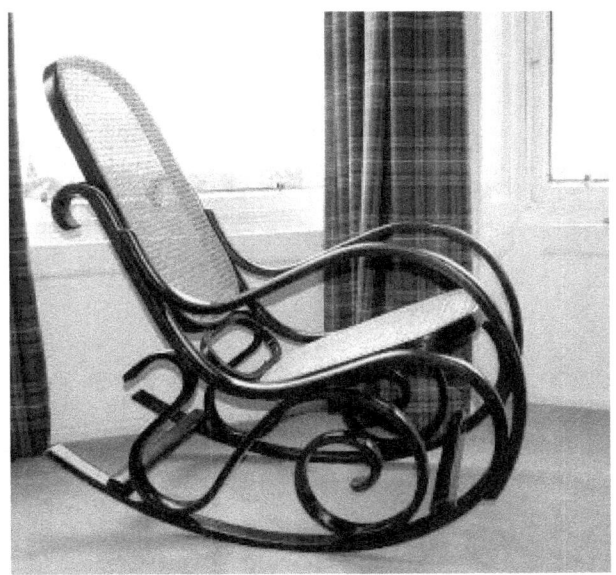

Avoiding Stress

Try Yoga, meditation, walking or deep breathing to reduce stress during your pregnancy, reducing stress will help you sleep better. Set aside 10-15 minutes during the day to sit in a quiet spot with refreshing drink ad your favorite music.

Don't forget to laugh once in a while, you'll feel better! Get together with friends who make you laugh, watch your favorite comedy show or movie or read a humorous book. Laughter is indeed the best medicine for many ailments as well as a great stress-reliever.

The stages of pregnancy

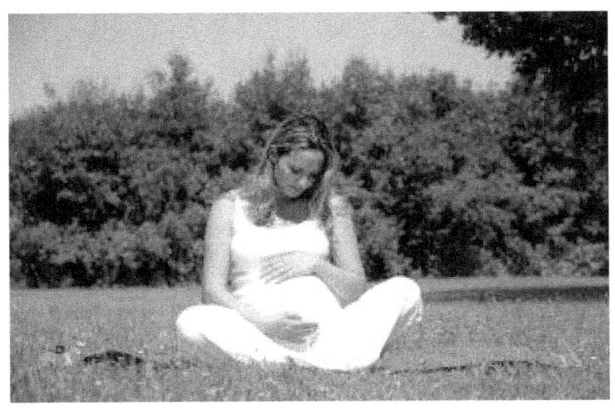

After the joy of finding out that you are pregnant, you want to know what changes your body will go through and what to expect. You also want to know what is happening to the baby growing inside you and the changes going on with him/her. The full term of pregnancy is divided into 3 trimester. You may have heard of trimesters but exactly happens in each phase?

Let's take a look at these three stages of pregnancy and talk about how your body changes and how your baby develops during these phases. Being aware of the potential changes will enable you to better take care of yourself and your unborn child during your pregnancy.

Tip: You or your husband can keep a journal of your pregnancy (including pictures) and record the changes you go through and how you are feeling week by week. Not only will it be great to read later on but will also be an invaluable record.

A normal pregnancy lasts about 40 weeks and is divided into three trimesters of three months each.

The first Trimester (Week 1 – week 12)

During this period your body undergoes many changes. Almost every organ in your body is affected by hormonal changes, and these changes can trigger certain symptoms as we discussed previously. One such these symptoms for example is your period stopping, is a clear sign that you are pregnant.

Other symptoms may include:

- Fatigue.

- Tender, swollen breasts.

- Morning sickness with or without vomiting.

- Headache.

- Heartburn.

- Mood swings.

As discussed earlier, there are ways to alleviate these discomforts. You will have to make changes to your daily routine as your body changes such as eating more frequently during the day, going to bed early or taking a nap in the afternoon.

Medical exams during the first trimester:

On your visit to your doctor after your pregnancy has been confirmed, He will first review your medical history and will do a range of tests to check your overall health. These tests include weight, blood pressure, and a pelvic exam.

He will also do blood tests in order to determine your blood type, and check for any diseases such as HIV. A urine test will be done to screen for diabetes or kidney problems.

Your baby in the first trimester

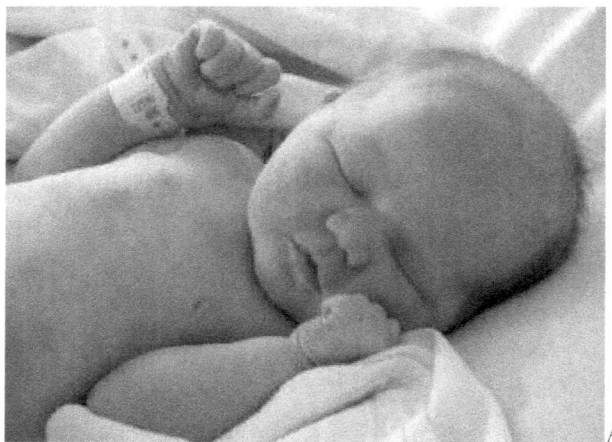

Although still very tiny, your baby in the first trimester us going through a lot of changes, too! He will have developed a heartbeat and tiny, moving limbs!

At four weeks:

- -Your baby's heart begins to form.

- The baby's arm and leg buds appear.

- Your baby's spinal cord and brain have begun to form.

- The baby is .25 inches long and is now an embryo.

- At Eight Weeks:

- Your baby will have a face!

- Toes and fingers have begun to form.

- Arms and legs grow longer.

- The external body structures and all major body organs have begun to form.

- The umbilical cord becomes clearly visible.

- The sex organs begin to form.

- The vital organs start to develop.

- At the end of these eight weeks your baby is a fetus and is one inch long.

Make sure your spouse or partner attends the very first ultrasound for your baby. It is one of the most thrilling and emotional experiences a human being can ever have

At Twelve weeks:

- The external sex organs show if the baby is a boy or a girl. You can find out the baby's sex if you have an ultrasound in the second trimester or later.

- Eyelids close in order to protect the developing eye; they will not open again until the 28th week.

- The baby is much longer now; it is about three inches long.

Tips for staying healthy in your first trimester:

- Stick to a healthy diet; eat several small meals instead of eating three big meals.

- Take your prenatal vitamins.

- Get plenty of sleep.

- Cut out smoking, drugs, and alcohol.

●

The Second Trimester (Week 14 -28)

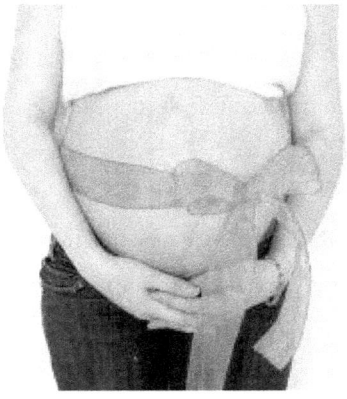

Say goodbye to nausea and morning sickness!

Most women find this trimester easier than the first. Symptoms like nausea and fatigue begin to fade while other noticeable, new changes to your body start to happen.

Many women suffer congestion during this period which can often be so severe that it causes snoring at night. If you suffer with this symptom and find it particularly bothersome, consult your doctor. He may prescribe a nasal decongestant spray.

You will start to feel your baby moving at the end of this trimester!

Changes that happen to your body during this period may be accompanied by the following symptoms:

- Body aches, such as back, thigh, or abdomen pain.

- Patches of darker skin which usually appear over the cheeks, nose, or upper lips, sometimes called the "mask of pregnancy." It has been found that dark-skinned women are more prone to this condition that fair-skinned women. This is due to the increase od Melanin in your body, a substance which causes skin and hair pigmentation. In most cases, these darker patches disappear within a few months after giving birth.

- Stretch marks appear on your abdomen, thighs, or breasts. This is a real horror for women. In some women they are barely noticeable, in others they are very pronounced. In most cases, stretch marks will gradually fade. Rubbing cocoa butter into these areas will also help, while giving our baby a comforting massage!

- Numb or tingling hands (Carpal Tunnel Syndrome).

- Swelling of the fingers, ankles, and face.

- Inflammation of the gums.

- Itching on the abdomen, palms, and feet. If this symptom is accompanied by nausea, vomiting, loss of appetite, or fatigue combined with itching, then you have to consult your doctor immediately because these could be signs of serious liver problems.

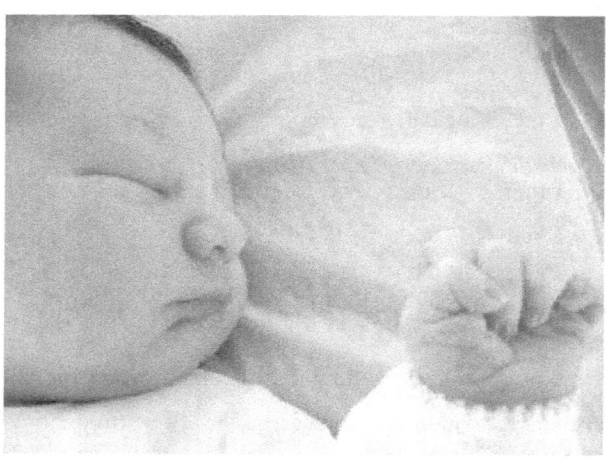

Your baby in the second trimester

At 16 weeks:

- -Skin begins to form.

- A substance called Meconium develops in the baby's intestinal tract, and this will form the first bowel movement of the baby.

- Your baby develops sucking reflex, where it starts to make sucking motions with the mouth, and may even suck is own thumb!

- The baby grows to a length of about four to five inches.

- Bones and muscle tissue begin to form.

At 20 weeks:

- The baby is covered in a waxy coating called Vernix, and by fine hair called Lanugo both of which protect the developing skin underneath.

- Eyelashes, fingernails, toenails, and eyebrows, have formed!

- The baby can hear and swallow. This is a great time for you and your spouse to begin talking to your baby – yes, he can hear you! Scientific observation as shown that babies hear and respond mostly to the mother's voice but can also distinguish other voices.

When talking to your baby, lean your face close to your belly, as the sound has to pass through several layers to get to him. Speak to your baby in a soft, soothing voice – scientific observation as actually shown that this has a calming, soothing effect on your baby and actually lows down the heart rate.

You can also read to your baby! Since unborn babies can hear inflection and cadence, choose children's books with a sing-son rhythm or rhyming words – Dr. Suess books are a great choice. This will also soothe your baby.

By the way… your baby is about six inches long now.

- At 24 Weeks:

- Taste buds are formed on the baby's tongue.

- Real hair begins to grow on the baby's head.

- The lungs are formed but don't work.

- Bone marrow starts to make blood cells.

- Footprints and fingerprints are formed.

- The baby is now about 12 inches long.

The Third Trimester (week 29-week 40)

In this stage some of the same discomforts that you have experienced in the second trimester will continue, plus new additional discomforts, where lots of women find breathing difficult, and notice that they have to go to the bathroom more frequently. and that is because as the baby grows bigger, it's putting more pressure on your organs, including the lungs and bladder.

Some symptoms of new body changes in the third trimester include:

- Heartburn.

- Hemorrhoids which are varicose veins in the rectal area. These may appear as a result of constipation - passing hard stools or straining during bowel movements.

- Trouble sleeping troubles. In many cases, the underlying cause may be fear of the impending labor and birth. Try herbal teas, meditaton or soothing music. A good night's sleep is essential to you in this phase so don't hesitate to inform your doctor of this problem.

- The baby gradually shifts and moves down lower in your belly.

- Contractions. These are most likely not labor contractions so don't panic. This will be discussed further a bit later and you will learn how to differentiate between "false" contractions and the real thing.

- Swelling of the fingers, face, and ankles.

Call your doctor immediately if you notice any extreme or sudden swelling, or if you gain a lot of weight very quickly, because this could be a sign of preeclampsia (High blood pressure during pregnancy).

As you get near your due date, your doctor will have to check your progress through a vaginal exam; your cervix becomes thinner and softer, which is a very normal process that helps the birth canal to open during birth.

Your baby in the third trimester

At 32 weeks:

- The baby's eyes can open and close and sense changes in the light.

- The baby's body starts to store vital minerals such as iron and calcium.

- The Lanugo starts to fall off in preparation for birth.

- The baby's bones are now completely formed, although still soft.

- The Lungs are still not completely formed.

- The baby is now 15-17 inches long.

At 36 weeks:

- The protective waxy coating called vernex becomes thicker.

- The baby is getting bigger, its movements are less forceful, but you will still feel wiggles and stretches.

- The baby is about 16-19 inches long.

At week 37-40:

- By the end of the 37 weeks, the baby's organs will be ready to function on their own, including the lungs.

- The baby will now be 19 to 21 inches long.

- The baby may now turn into a head-down position in preparation for birth, as you are very near your due date.

Tips for the third trimester:

This is the time to consider taking classes like childbirth classes, baby care classes, or breastfeeding classes.

Choose a pediatrician for your baby. It's good to know exactly where to go in case your baby gets ill, to avoid a panic. Ideally, you will stay with that pediatrician throughout your baby's first years and early childhood, so make sure you make a good choice.

Set up a safe place for your baby to sleep. If you haven't done so yet, shop for baby clothes, crib, bottles and other baby things to avoid a last-minute scramble

Continue to talk to your baby! Remember, he can hear you and this is the best way to start the bonding process.

At last - Your little miracle is ready to come into the world!

Be prepared –planning for your delivery

What is a birth plan?

The birth of your baby should be one of the most joyful and memorable experiences of your life and taking the time to prepare a birth plan will help to ensure that.

A birth plan is a document that gives your medical team information about your preferences during the delivery as well as important topics to discuss with your delivery team. It includes things such as how to manage labor pain, whether you prefer a natural birth or a medically assisted birth (epidural)…In short, it is a way for you to communicate your hopes and wishes to the doctors who care for you during your labor and delivery. It also gives them an idea about the type of birth and labor you'd like to have.

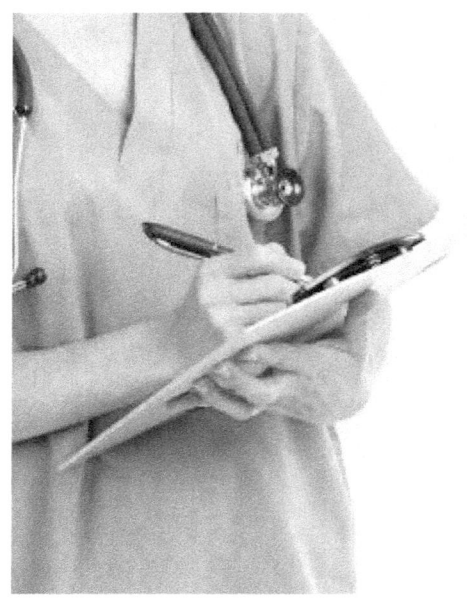

A birth plan is not set in stone; it has to be flexible in order to accommodate any last minute changes, medical or otherwise.

You will have to stay flexible in case anything comes up that requires your birth team to depart from your plan because of course you will not be able to control every aspect of labor and delivery. For example in case an emergency arises your preferences will have to be overridden for the sake of your own or your baby's safety.

Write a plan that doesn't make your doctor feel that his hands are tied in case complications arise during labor. A birth plan can also inform new members of your medical team about your preferences while you are in active labor, and will also refresh your provider's memory at that time.

Mutual cooperation and respect between you and your delivery team will guarantee the best outcome.

Tips for making the ideal birth plan:

- Your birth plan should ideally be a simple, clear, one-page document stating your preferences for you and your child

- Make sure to write details about your medical history in your birth plan.

- If you have had a baby before, make sure to include any past experiences/complications that may affect this birth.

- State what kinds of pain relief - if any -you would like to receive and in what order. For instance, you may prefer to use Pethidine before an epidural. Also make sure to write down any types of pain relief you would like to avoid using.

- Mention if you would like your doctor to intervene to speed up your labor if it slows down, or if you would prefer to wait and see what happens naturally.

- Mention whether you would like your baby to be placed directly on your stomach straight after birth or whether you prefer that your baby is cleaned up first before it is handed to you.

- Write down what you want to happen if your baby has to go to the special care baby unit (SCBU).

- Make sure to mention whether or not you will need an interpreter in case English is not your first language.

- Include any religious requirements you would like to be carried out when your baby is born.

- Mention if you will need a special diet during your hospital stay.

Most hospitals provide a birth plan brochure that explains the hospital's philosophy on childbirth; you can use this birth plan brochure to note your preferences. Make sure to give a copy to your provider and to the nurses at the hospital.

You can also find examples of birthing plans on different parenting websites. I have found an excellent very detailed birth plan on this website that is free to print out and use:

http://www.earthmamaangelbaby.com/free-birth-plan

What happens after you've written your plan?

Show your birth plan to your doctor to confirm that the and the hospital staff will be able to comply with your wishes. Discussing your plan will give you a chance to ask questions, and learn more about will happen during your delivery.

Considerations for your delivery

When making plans for your delivery, you should consider the location of the delivery, and whether you will need labor support from your spouse, a friend, or family members and get this arranged.

Childbirth education classes

You should also decide whether you will attend a childbirth education class, and if so you should start during your sixth or seventh month of pregnancy.

What will you learn in a childbirth education class?

A childbirth class is an excellent option to prepare for labor and birth, especially for first-time mothers. Although the methods may vary from class to class, the goal is the same: to prepare you for labor and delivery, ease your fears regarding labor and help you make informed decisions when the big event finally arrives.

Most childbirth classes also address common complications and how they should be handled. You will learn breathing techniques help you cope with labor pains as well as pre-birth exercises to help facilitate the delivery.

There are different types of birth of childbirth classes and we will give you a brief idea about each:

The famous Lamaze, technique widely popular in the U.S. This method focuses mainly on breathing technique and building up a mother's confidence in preparation for childbirth.

The Bradley Method, also known as the husband-coached method. This method focuses on preparing the mother-to-be to give birth completely naturally without any drugs. It relies on the presence of the spouse or partner to "coach" the woman through labor. Needless to say, this is a class that must be attended by the couple.

Hypnobirthing : Hypnotherapy for pregnant mothers is fairly new to the scene but has been quickly gaining ground. This is a fairly new method and focuses on preparation for childbirth and painless childbirth through self-hypnosis. They also teach various methods of prenatal bonding between mother and child.

Hospital childbirth preparation classes: These types of classes are quite traditional but the quality can vary from one hospital to another. They teach basic anatomy, the stages of labor, breathing techniques and hospital childbirth procedures.

Birth Works: This method is also fairly knew to the scene. It is perhaps the first childbirth preparation class that deals in depth with the emotional preparation for birth as well as the physical. Their flyer states: *"Birth Works embodies a philosophy that develops a woman's self-confidence and trust in her innate ability to give birth. The classes are experimental and provide both a physical and emotional preparation for birth."* This is an ideal class for women who are planning a home birth.

Although the methods may differ, the majority of childbirth classes cover the following topics:

- Signs of labor

- The progress of labor and the birth.

- Techniques and exercises to minimize and cope with pain.

- How your partner can assist and support you during labor

- General complications.

- Cesarean birth versus vaginal birth

- Some classes also include the basics of how to care for you newborn baby.

- Some classes may cover breastfeeding.

Most hospitals and various childbirth organizations offer childbirth preparation classes - including your local hospital, most likely. This may be the easiest and most affordable option for you. New mothers in particular will find them very helpful in learning about labor and delivery ahead of time, and being informed about how to handle the first hours with your newborn.

Home Delivery?

Since the beginning of time, before hospitals and birth centers, women all over the world gave birth at home, whether "home" was a cave, a hut, a medieval palace or a 16th century manor house. In fact, up until the 1920s, all women gave birth at home.

Many women today are opting to "go back to their roots" and give birth at home. They prefer to deliver their babies at home, in the comfort of their own bed amidst familiar surroundings, with family members and friends close by.

If you are a healthy expectant mother, your pregnancy is progressing smoothly and your doctor foresees no complications, a home birth can be an option for you.

A home birth is overseen by a qualified midwife and is completely natural – no pain medications, no epidural, no hospital staff interruptions and can be attended by as many friends and family members as you want. Note that if you do opt for a home birth, prepare to be flexible should complications arise; in such a case you will have to be taken to hospital. Today, a homebirth that is carefully monitored by a skilled practitioner is very safe for a woman who has been shown to be low-risk.

Many women swear by home births while others throw their hands up in horror at the idea, preferring the sterile hospital environment and a trained medical team on hand. Both options are fine; the choice depends on your specific mindset and preferences.

The Cesarean birth

A C-section is the delivery of the child through an incision in the mother's uterus. In some circumstances, the procedure may be scheduled in advanced for certain health reasons, or sometimes even planned by the mother herself. In other cases it may be done as an emergency procedure due to unforeseen complications during the birth.

You may require a planned C-section if:

- You have had a previous C-section with a vertical incision or more than one previous C-section, as there is a risk of rupture of your uterus if you have a vaginal delivery.

- If you have had any other kind of uterine surgery.

- If your baby is very large.

- If your baby is in a breech position (bottom downwards instead of head) or transverse(sideways).

- If you are carrying more than one baby. In some cases twins can be delivered vaginally but more than that will require a C-section.

You may need to have an unplanned (emergency) C-section if:

- Your baby stops moving down the birth canal

- Your cervix stops dilating.

- The umbilical cord slips through your cervix. This may cause oxygen to be cut off from your baby.

- Your baby's heart rate slows down or weakens, a sign that he may not be able to withstand prolonged labor.

- If your placenta separates from the uterine wall, cutting off the baby's oxygen supply.

Some women also plan C-sections of their own accord to avoid the discomforts of labor. This trend has increased dramatically in modern times.

Planning for Breastfeeding

The American Academy of Pediatrics recommends breastfeeding due to its many benefits for you and your child. If you are able to breastfeed your newborn and are considering this as an option, here are some of the wonderful benefits to be gained:

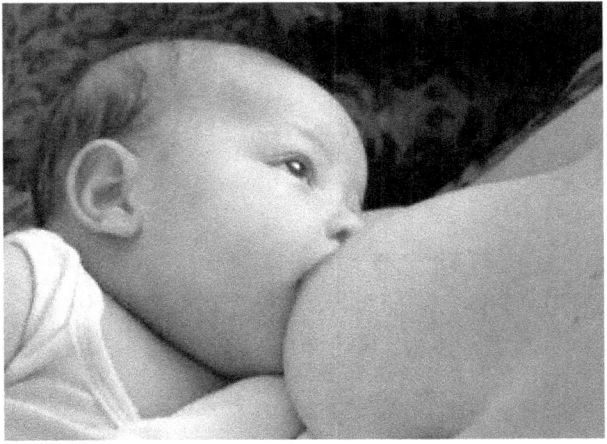

Protects your baby from numerous illnesses: Studies from across the globe have shown that babies who are breast have a lower risk of contracting stomach viruses, ear infections and meningitis as well as many other diseases and infections.

Boosts your baby's immunity: The first milk the flows from your breasts contains a substance called secretory immunoglobulin A (IgA) which is present in large amounts. It continues to be present in moderate amounts in your breast milk after that. This substance has been shown to boost immunity in the child and make him more resistance to contracting diseases and infections.

Protects your baby from developing allergies: Studies have shown that babies who are breastfed are less likely to develop allergies. They believe this is due to the immunity boosting substances in breast milk

Protects your baby from obesity: Breastfed babies have been shown to have more Lepin in their system, a hormone that regulates appetite.

Babies who are breast fed are 4 to 5 times less likely to develop diarrheal disease.

Nursing mothers are less likely to develop osteoporosis.

Breastfeeding helps a mother to lose weight more easily after giving birth.

The risk of contracting breast cancer is reduced by 24% in women who breastfeed for more than 2 years and also decreases the risk of ovarian cancer.

The emotional health of both mother and child benefits from the special bond that develops between them during breastfeeding.

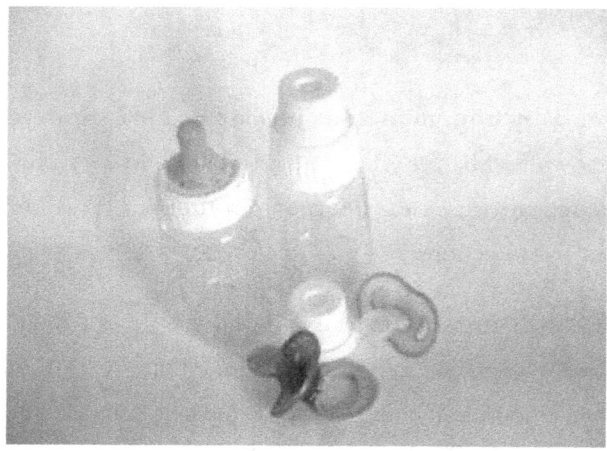

Plan for breastfeeding ahead of time!

Learn more about breastfeeding, find a good lactation consultant early and buy necessary supplies such as nursing bras, towels, etc.

Decide whether you want to hold your baby after birth and breast feed immediately, or not (This can be included in your birth plan).

Decide how you feel about the use of a pacifier or bottles in between breast feedings.

Packing and final preparation for delivery

Pack your suitcase in advance in order to ensure that you have everything you'll need during delivery.

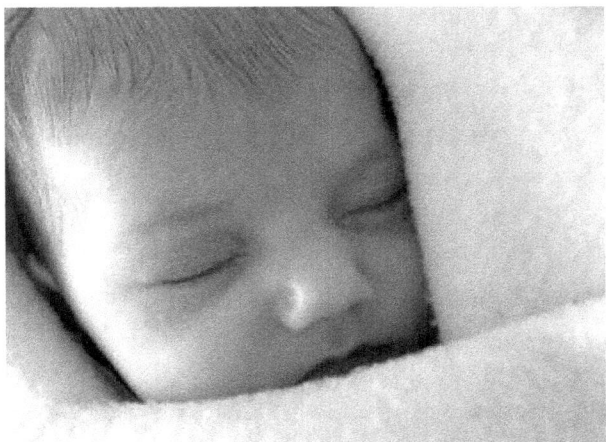

Make sure to put in your suitcase:

- Hair clips or bands which will help keep your hair out of the way.

- Soothing music or tapes for relaxation.

- Take gowns, slippers, and a bathrobe for the hospital, and a loose – fitting outfit to wear home.

- If you are nursing, take nursing bras and gowns.

- Also pack clothes and blankets for the baby's trip home.

- Photos and magazines will help pass the time.

- Socks to keep your feet warm.

Don't forget to stock up on frozen food ahead of time so that you can focus on taking care of your baby for the first week or two when you return home.

Plan for the transportation you will take to the facility where you will give birth, and try to get more information about the parking procedures, and which entrance you can use in case you arrive after hours.

A hospital is the best place to give birth in, and your doctor should advise you to give birth in a hospital if you have high risk pregnancy needs such as very early preterm labor where you will have to be admitted to a hospital with a high risk pregnancy service.

While most women prefer to a vaginal birth, other women with a low lying placenta or those with a baby in the breech position may be advised to have a caesarian section, as discussed previously

In case of a caesarian delivery, there will be some risk such as blood clots, infection, and excessive bleeding as with any surgical procedure. However, recovery is generally very quick and most C-sections are performed without complications.

Tips before delivery:

If you are feeling anxiety about giving birth, consider receiving therapy for your concerns, learning relaxation techniques such as breathing exercises or meditation would greatly help.

Talking things over with family members or other women who have experienced birth can help to ease your fears about delivery.

Remember: Healthy Mom and Healthy baby, that's the end result that we all want!

ELANE HOLLOWAY

The big day is finally here-what to do during labor

At last! You have finally reached the big day You're a bundle of mixed emotions: excitement, exhilaration, anticipation ... and fear The fear is normal and expected. In fact, it would be abnormal if you didn't feel at least a twinge of fear during this life-changing event. This chapter will give you some basic information about going into labor and what to expect.

Signs of labor:

You're probably unaware of this but your body actually starts preparing for labor about a month before you give birth. However, medical experts have been unable to pinpoint what exactly triggers a woman to go into labor and therefore no doctors is able to predict the exact date and time you will be ready to deliver your baby.

Here are some signs and symptoms you may experience as your due date draws near.

Your baby drops: This is where the baby moves lower in your womb and the head turns upside down in preparation for emerging into the world. will experience a feeling of heaviness in the pelvic area and more lightness in the area of your upper stomach and ribcage, making it easier for you to breathe.

Contractions: Just before birth these contractions will be felt to be more like menstrual cramps, setting the stage for real labor contractions.

Cervix dilation: This will be confirmed by your doctor who will do a pelvic exam and inform you that you will go into labor very soon.

Increased vaginal discharge, mucous or light bleeding: This is a sign that your cervix is dilation, and that the "mucous plug" that has sealed it during pregnancy is beginning to disintegrate. This plug may come out in one lump or in the form of increased vaginal discharge over several days before birth. This discharge may be ringed with some light-colored blood

Water breaking. This is the sign that the amniotic sac surrounding your baby has ruptured and is the most certain sign that your labor has started. When the water breaks it may come out in a large gush or a trickle. Both case are normal.

In most cases, the real contractions start after the water breaks. If contractions don't start within a certain amount of time, you may have to be induced as your baby may be at risk of infection.

When should you call your doctor or midwife after your water breaks?

Near the end of your term, your doctor or midwife will give you clear guidelines regarding the timing of your contractions and when o call him/her. Some health practitioners prefer an early head-up while others may want to wait until the contractions are coming a bit faster and lasting longer. You will then be instructed to proceed to the hospital or birth center.

Contractions during labor:

Labor contractions may range from discomfort and aching in your back and lower abdomen to outright pain. The way contractions feel is different from one woman to another and from one pregnancy to the next.

Contractions take place in the womb and are nature's method of pushing the baby out. They start at the top of the uterus to the bottom and resemble strong menstrual cramps. Changing your position or relaxing does not stop labor contractions.

Now let's discuss the terms mentioned previously in a little bit more detail.

Water breaking during labor

Water breaking could be just a slow trickle that is only enough to dampen your underwear or you may wake up to a wet sheet in the morning. In rare cases there will be a dramatic gush of water.

Inform your doctor immediately if the waters are smelly or colored, or if you are losing blood, because this could mean that you and your baby need urgent help.

Passing of the mucus plug

As mentioned earlier, this is one of the signs that you are very near to giving birth. During pregnancy, the mucus plug accumulates at the cervix; the mucus is discharged into the vagina when the cervix begins to open,

This mucus may be clear, pink, or slightly bloody.

Labor may begin just after the mucus plug is discharged, or one to two weeks later.

Lightening: This is the process of your baby settling in your pelvis just before labor.

Lightening can occur a few hours or a few weeks before labor, and at that time you may feel that you need to urinate more frequently and that is because your baby's head is pressing on your bowel.

False Labor

You may experience false labor pains also known as "Braxton Hicks contractions" before your real labor begins. These contractions are normal and usually begin in the second trimester, although they are more common in the third trimester of pregnancy.

What is the difference between true labor and false labor?

A sign that you are experiencing false labor is that Braxton Hicks contractions do not increase when walking, but actually may stop if you walk or rest. False contractions do not increase in duration and do not get stronger over time as they do during true labor.

False labor contractions are only felt in the front of the abdomen or pelvic region, where as true labor contractions usually start in the lower back and move to the front of the abdomen.

False labor contractions are usually weak and do not get stronger or they may be strong at first and then get weaker, whereas true labor contractions steadily increase in strength and duration.

When is it an emergency?

You should contact your doctor immediately if:

- Your baby is moving less than usual or has stopped moving completely.

- Your waters break and contractions don't start within an hour afterwards.

- You have vaginal bleeding.

- You have severe headaches, changes in your vision or a fever accompanied by abdominal pain.

What you should do early on in labor

The first thing to do is to keep calm and relaxed. It's the moment you've been waiting for. Any pain or discomfort will soon be over and forgotten and you'll be holding your little bundle of joy arms. Do some deep breathing or meditation; it will help your body release the hormone called oxytocin which you will need for your labor to progress, or do anything else that will help you to stay relaxed such as going for a walk, watching a film you like… try taking a warm shower to ease pains, or ask a close friend or relative over to keep you company until it's time to go to the hospital.

Your spouse or partner can also rub your back as this can help relieve pain.

As the contractions get stronger, you can try breathing exercises.

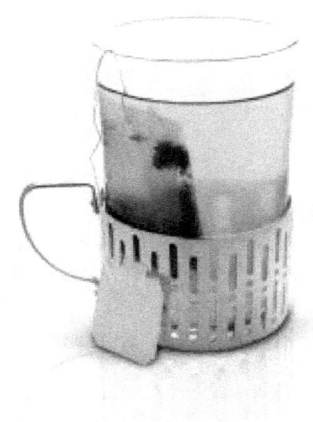

Staying hydrated is important for a mother in labor, as lack of fluids can weaken you. In the past, women in labor were not supposed to eat or drink and many people still hold to that practice – wrong! There's no harm whatsoever in eating and drinking during childbirth. You can drink moderate amounts of water, isotronic drinks to keep your body nourished, raspberry leaf tea, ginger tea, or coconut water. All are ideal for a laboring mother.

Eat healthy but light foods like protein, vegetables, or fruit.

Make sure your bags are packed and ready to go.

Finally, that your mindset is very important for the stage of labor. Fear heightens pain during labor, so avoid pregnancy books and classes that over-hype the pain of labor. More importantly, avoid listening to friends who are eager to tell you their horror stories about their own deliveries. Don't be shy to cut them off mid-sentence. If they're not tactful enough to avoid scaring you, you don't need to be polite.

Labor doesn't have to be terrifying, so don't live in fear of it while you are pregnant. When a woman tells you she was in labor for 40 hours, you can bet she's counting from the early stages of labor—not hard labor. Don't let tales like this one worry you.

If it was really that horrible why do so many women willingly get pregnant several times over?

If you feel you need more information about labor, a childbirth class will arm you with lots of knowledge. The amazing World Wide Web is also a great source of information. You can find dozens of great websites for expectant mothers that will give as much detailed information as you need.

Remember to stay fit!

Continue to Swim, walk, take a prenatal exercise class or any other form of exercise as previously discussed - after getting an O.K from your doctor, of course.

Pregnant women who stay in shape usually have shorter labors.

Hey Dad!

The birth of a child is one of the most miraculous and incredible experiences you will ever get to be a part of, and sharing the experience of pregnancy and childbirth with your partner will bond you together even more. Make sure you're available to share her joy, fears, worried and that incredible moment when your child is born.

Of course, there's no way a man can fully comprehend what it feels like to carry baby to full term and all the changes that accompany that – but there are ways to participate:

Be an "active observer": Show your spouse or partner that you are enjoying the pregnancy by feeling the baby kick, playing music and reading to it.

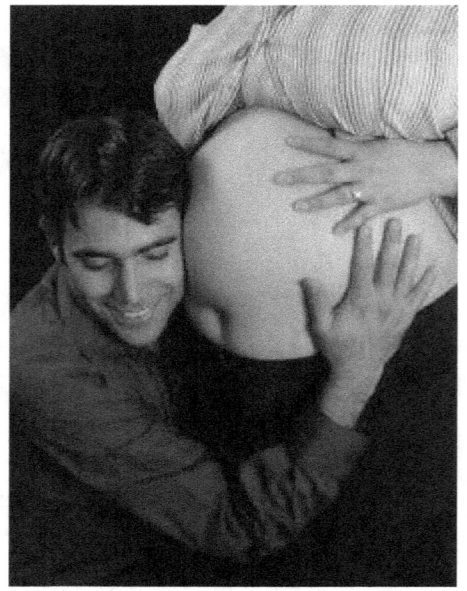

Record the memories: Start a scrapbook/ journal in which you record the events of the pregnancy, complete with photos of your spouse during the various stages. It's not quite common for many husbands to videotape the birth itself!

Give reassurance: Your spouse's pregnancy will not be smooth sailing all the way. There will be times when she has fears and worries; be there to calm those fears and reassure her that everything will be fine. As she grows bigger she will feel clumsy and unattractive; tell her you've never seen her more beautiful; she may not feel like having sex as frequently as you used to; grin and bear it.

Get educated: You can never really know what's like to be pregnant. But learning about the stages of pregnancy and the physical and emotional changes that a woman through will help you understand what your wife is experiencing.

Share in the preparations – Go shopping with your partner for maternity clothes, and later when you know the sex of your baby, shop together for baby clothes. Help her decorate the baby's room and spend an evening or two discussing possible baby names.

Get into shape: Encourage your spouse to maintain a healthy lifestyle by joining her at her exercise routine. Help her prepare healthy meals and enjoy them together.

Become a hero in your partner's eyes by learning how to change a diaper.

Be there: Try to make yourself available for your partner's doctor appointments. Seeing your baby during the ultrasound or finding out the baby's sex is an event not to be missed!

Your job in the first stage of labor is to keep yourself and your partner calm, try relaxation exercises, a massage, or go for a short walk together, if you can't stick around for too long make sure to be always available when your partner says "it's time".

Your role in the hospital is important and is sure to put a big, appreciative smile on her face:

Keep your hand handy! Be prepared to get your hand squeezed to death while she's in labor. Stroke her head and be generous with words of comfort.

Be on hand to hold the baby if she needs to use the bathroom or shower.

Buy her flowers to keep at her bedside.

Be ready to run out for sandwiches, snacks or last minute items for her or the baby.

Sit down, take break, take out your mobile and share the good news on Twitter or Facebook!

Some more tips for the dad-to-be

Keep the doctor/midwife's number handy for when your partner's labor starts.

Memorize the route to the hospital.

Be informed about the hospital parking system.

If you're driving, keep the gas tank full as her due date nears.

Make sure you have a copy of the birth plan.

If you're planning to film the birth, make sure your camera/cell phone is charged.

Remain calm and in control!

Finally, face your fears. The reason why so many men seem detached from the whole process is fear: What is something goes wrong during the birth? What if the baby is not born perfect? Will you be able to love your new baby? If you don't have these fears you wouldn't be normal. Talk to friends or relative who are dads; they will be able to reassure you.

Summary and general tips

- Delivering a baby is a very natural event and should not be considered an illness although it requires medication and surgery.

-Give your baby the best chance to start a healthy life by eating right, exercising, and making any necessary life style changes you may need.

-Put in mind that every pregnancy is different, and that every labor and delivery is also different.

-Prenatal vitamins are essential not only for your health but also for your baby's health.

- It's better to start taking prenatal vitamins before you get that positive pregnancy test.

-Folic acid is a key ingredient in prenatal vitamins, as it can prevent birth defects such as Spinal Bifida and Cleft Palate.

-If you choose to breast feed, it's very important for you to seek help before the baby comes.

-Eating healthy foods during pregnancy is the most important thing; you need more protein, iron, calcium, and folic acid than you did before pregnancy.

-The best recipe for good health during pregnancy is eating sensible balanced meals together with regular physical fitness.

-Weight gain during pregnancy:

The amount of weight you should gain during pregnancy depends on your weight before you got pregnant. Remember that eating for two does not mean eating twice as much.

-If you were underweight before pregnancy then you should gain between 28-40 pounds during pregnancy. If you were overweight before pregnancy then you should gain between 15-25 pounds during pregnancy.

- If you were at normal weight before pregnancy then you should gain between 25-30 pounds during pregnancy. If you were obese before pregnancy then you should gain between 11-20 pounds during pregnancy.

-Studies show that gaining more weight than the recommended during pregnancy may raise your child's chances of being overweight in the future.

-Make sure to clean, and cool food properly in order to prevent food borne illness such as Listeria, and Toxoplasmosis.

-Keep raw meats and seafood from touching other foods or surfaces.

-Wash cooking pans with hot, soapy water.

-Wash your hands with soap before touching soil, or raw meat.

-Avoid eating:

- Unpasteurized milk or juices.

- Unpasteurized soft cheese such as blue cheese.

- Fish with high levels of mercury such as tile fish, shark, or king mackerel. *Mercury is a metal that at high levels may harm the brain of your unborn baby.*

- Refrigerated smoked seafood such as salmon, or whitefish.

-Check before eating fish found in local waters; remember that state health departments have guidelines on fish from local waters.

-Never use herbs and plants as medicines without consulting your doctor, as they may be very harmful during pregnancy.

-Don't forget fluids during pregnancy! Remember that your body needs more water to stay hydrated and support the baby inside you.

-Water also helps prevent constipation, excessive swelling, hemorrhoids, and urinary tract and bladder infections during pregnancy.

-Remember that your body will need more fluids when in hot weather, when you have a fever, or if you have diarrhea, or if you are vomiting.

-It is recommended that pregnant women drink 10 cups of fluid daily including coffee, tea, water, juices, and soft drinks.

-You can check if your fluid intake is O.K. by checking the color of your urine, it should be pale yellow or colorless. *Don't wait until you feel thirsty to drink. Thirst is a sign that your body is on its way to dehydration, which is very dangerous during pregnancy.*

-Avoid drinking Alcohol during pregnancy; the alcohol in your blood reaches your baby's body through the umbilical cord, which can affect your baby's brain, cause birth defects, and slow down your baby's growth.

-Moderate amounts of caffeine such as less than 200 mg of caffeine per day appear to be safe during pregnancy; some studies have shown that higher amounts of caffeine may increase the risk of miscarriage, and preterm birth, but there is no solid proof about that.

- Keep fit!

-Physical fitness during pregnancy helps keep the heart, bones, and mind healthy.

-Active women are better prepared for labor and delivery and recover more quickly.

-Staying active by exercising protects your emotional health, and puts you at a lower risk of depression and anxiety.

-Pregnant women who are physically active may lower their chances of preterm delivery.

- Exercising prevents pains and aches during pregnancy including backaches, and constipation.

-Consult your doctor before exercising because he may advise you not to exercise if you have any of the following conditions:

- Vaginal bleeding.
- Premature rupture of membranes that is if your water breaks early before labor.
- Risks for preterm labor.

Best activities for the moms-to-be:

-The best activities for women during pregnancy are low impact activities, such as walking, swimming, dancing, and low impact aerobics.

-Avoid activities in which you can get hit in the abdomen such as soccer or basketball.

-Avoid activities in which you can fall such as horseback riding, and gymnastics.

-Avoid scuba diving as it can create gas bubbles in your baby's blood which can cause many health problems.

-When you exercise you have to start slowly, progress gradually, and cool down slowly.

-Don't do any exercise on your back during your first trimester, as this can put pressure on an important vein in your body and prevent blood flow to your baby.

-Be careful, try not to lose your balance and remember that your centre of gravity has changed which makes you more prone to falls.

Oral Health:

-Before you become pregnant make sure to take good care of your gums and teeth and keep them healthy, so it's best to

 Have dental checkups routinely.

-Have a complete oral exam early in your pregnancy, so that if you are in need of an x-ray for the treatment of any dental problem you may have it while the health risk during using x-rays to your unborn baby is small.

-Dental treatment during pregnancy is safe and the best times for treatment is between the 14th and 20th week, you might feel uncomfortable sitting in a dentist chair during the last months of pregnancy!

Traveling during pregnancy

-Everyday life doesn't have to stop once you are pregnant, you can continue with your routine and activity level such as working and traveling.

-Make sure to talk to your doctor if you plan on traveling and be sure to consider the destination, will there be good medical care available in case of any emergency, is the food and water safe.

-Avoid sitting for long periods during car or air travel, take frequent breaks to stretch your legs.

-If you get any problems with your pregnancy during your trip, don't wait until you go back home, seek medical care right away.

Environmental risks

-Avoid exposure to substances that might put your health or your unborn baby's health at risk, such as:

-Mercury: The harmful form is found mainly in large predatory fish.

-Solvents: Such as paint strippers and thinners.

-Cigarette smoke.

-Lead: Found in some water and paints.

-Arsenic: High levels may be found in some well waters.

Put in mind that you can never predict how much exposure can lead to problems such as miscarriage or birth defects, so the best thing to do is to avoid or limit your exposure as much as possible.

The following are some simple day-to-day precautions that you can take:

-Do not clean the inside of an oven during your pregnancy.

-Leave the house if paints are being use.

-Open the windows or use a fan while you are cleaning.

Smoking:

-Quit smoking immediately! Smoking can be very harmful to your health and your baby's health.

-Smoking during pregnancy increases the risk of low birth weight babies, or sudden infant death syndrome (SIDS).

Illegal drugs

-Avoid using illegal drugs during pregnancy because this could be very dangerous, especially to those women who inject drugs whom will be at a higher risk of catching HIV, which can be passed to an unborn baby.

ELANE HOLLOWAY

When to call your doctor

Call your doctor immediately if you:

- Have sudden or severe swelling in the face, hands, or fingers.

- Have vaginal bleeding.

- Have a fever or chills.

- Have problems seeing or blurred vision.

- Feel dizzy.

- Have depression and are thinking of harming yourself or your baby.

- Have pain or cramping in your lower abdomen.

- Suspect that your baby is moving less than normal and that is if you count less than 10 movements within two hours.

Remember that if you are a victim of abuse or violence from someone you know or love, you and your baby can get immediate support.

Get all the rest you can, sleep well and be calm; you will need it after that little bundle of joy enters your life.

ELANE HOLLOWAY

Myths about childbirth and pregnancy.

To end on a light note, check out these myths about childbirth and pregnancy and have a good chuckle!

Myth: A high baby bump means it's a girl, a low baby bump means it's a boy.

Fact: Totally untrue. This myth obviously went into circulation before ultrasound was invented!

Myth: You're eating for two.

Fact: Not so fast – don't start gorging yourself silly on ice cream and pie. A healthy pregnant mother only needs 300 extra calories a day, equivalent to a glass of skimmed milk and half a sandwich.

Myth: Avoid hair dyes and perms.

Fact: Hair dyes and perming solutions do not contain enough chemicals to harm your baby in any way. In fact, a new hair color may be a great pick-me-up during those "low" times in your pregnancy.

Myth: If you suffer from heartburn during pregnancy, your baby will be born with a full head of hair.

Fact: No comment.

Myth: If you have a craving for a certain food and don't satisfy it, your baby will look like that food.

Fact: I know a woman who resisted a craving for lobster. Her baby look perfectly human.

Myth: If your face is round and rosy, you're having a girl.

Fact: All expectant mothers radiate with a special glow during pregnancy regardless of the baby's sex.

Myth: Don't stay mad at someone while you're pregnant or your baby will look like that person.

Fact: I guess this was before DNA was discovered.

Myth: Drinking orange juice will cause you to miscarry but eating oranges will not.

Fact: Where does orange juice come from?

Conclusion

Having a baby is a miraculous and exciting journey. A child is a blessing, a gift from God and an event to celebrate no matter what your circumstances are.

Hopefully, this book has given you the basic information you need to help you through your pregnancy and calm any apprehensions you may have had your pregnancy with all its ups and downs, try to relax and enjoy every moment. Before you know it, you will be looking down into your child's tiny angelic face and realize that you have performed a miracle. That's something that no book can prepare you for.

Best wishes for a safe delivery and a beautiful son/daughter!

ELANE HOLLOWAY

ABOUT THE AUTHOR

Elane Holloway has spent her life with children. She has been a nanny, worked in day care centers, guided women through their pregnancies, assisted in countless deliveries as a Douala, and has raised her own children for all of their lives. She specializes in counseling women on raising children through their formative years.

She was born and raised in Michigan and lives in the Detroit area with her husband, two children, and their cat, Motzart. Incidentally, she is also a avid Dr. Who fan.

www.ingramcontent.com/pod-product-compliance
Lightning Source LLC
Chambersburg PA
CBHW060637290526
45793CB00001B/287